The Healthy Dash Diet Collection

How To Burn Your Calories Quickly

Candace Hickman

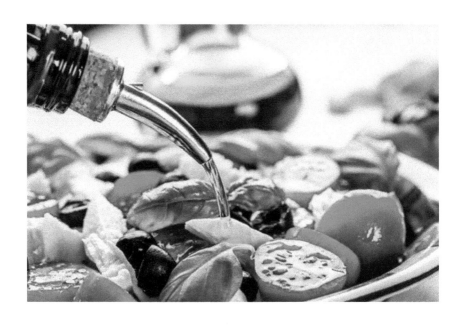

TABLE OF CONTENT

Spiced Chicken Mix

Preparation time: 10 minutes

Cooking time: 30 minutes

Servings: 4

Ingredients:

- 1 pound chicken breast, skinless, boneless and sliced
- 4 scallions, chopped
- 1 tablespoon olive oil
- 1 tablespoon sweet paprika
- 1 cup low-sodium chicken stock
- 1 tablespoon ginger, grated
- 1 teaspoon oregano, dried
- 1 teaspoon cumin, ground
- 1 teaspoon allspice, ground
- ½ cup cilantro, chopped
- A pinch of black pepper

Directions:

1. Heat up a pan with the oil over medium heat, add the scallions and the meat and brown for 5 minutes.

2. Add the rest of the ingredients, toss, introduce in the oven and bake at 390 degrees F for 25 minutes.
3. Divide the chicken and scallions mix between plates and serve.

Nutrition info per serving: 180 calories, 25.1g protein, 3.9g carbohydrates, 6.9g fat, 1.6g fiber, 73mg cholesterol, 97mg sodium, 551mg potassium

Mustard Chicken

Preparation time: 10 minutes

Cooking time: 35 minutes

Servings: 4

Ingredients:

- 1 pound chicken thighs, boneless and skinless
- 1 tablespoon avocado oil
- 2 tablespoons mustard
- 1 shallot, chopped
- 1 cup low-sodium chicken stock
- 3 garlic cloves, minced
- ½ teaspoon basil, dried

Directions:

1. Heat up a pan with the oil over medium heat, add the shallot, garlic and the chicken and brown everything for 5 minutes.
2. Add the mustard and the rest of the ingredients, toss gently, bring to a simmer and cook over medium heat for 30 minutes.
3. Divide everything between plates and serve hot.

Nutrition info per serving: 253 calories, 34.7g protein, 3.3g carbohydrates, 10.5g fat, 1g fiber, 101mg cholesterol, 132mg sodium, 343mg potassium

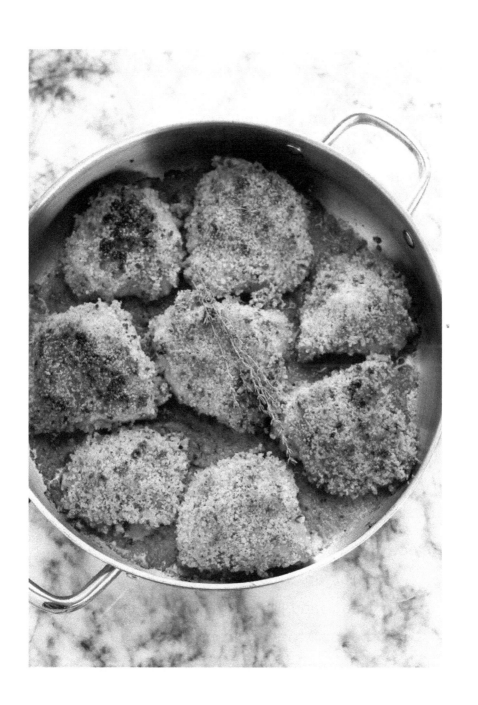

Chili Chicken Mix

Preparation time: 10 minutes

Cooking time: 35 minutes

Servings: 4

Ingredients:

- A pinch of black pepper
- 2 pounds chicken breast, skinless, boneless and cubed
- 2 tablespoons olive oil
- 1 cup celery, chopped
- 3 garlic cloves, minced
- 1 poblano pepper, chopped
- 1 cup low-sodium vegetable stock
- 1 teaspoon chili powder
- 2 tablespoons chives, chopped

Directions:

1. Heat up a pan with the oil over medium heat, add the garlic, celery and poblano pepper, toss and cook for 5 minutes.
2. Add the meat, toss and cook for another 5 minutes.

3. Add the rest of the ingredients except the chives, bring to a simmer and cook over medium heat for 25 minutes more.
4. Divide the whole mix between plates and serve with the chives sprinkled on top.

Nutrition info per serving: 338 calories, 49g protein, 4g carbohydrates, 12.9g fat, 1.1g fiber, 145mg cholesterol, 179mg sodium, 1001mg potassium

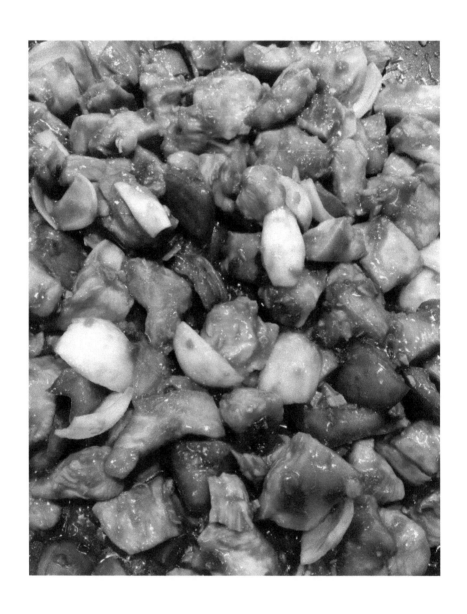

Turkey and Potatoes

Preparation time: 10 minutes

Cooking time: 40 minutes

Servings: 4

Ingredients:

- 1 turkey breast, skinless, boneless and sliced
- 2 tablespoons olive oil
- 1 pound baby potatoes, peeled and halved
- 1 tablespoon sweet paprika
- 1 yellow onion, chopped
- 1 teaspoon chili powder
- 1 teaspoon rosemary, dried
- 2 cups low-sodium chicken stock
- A pinch of black pepper
- Zest of 1 lime, grated
- 1 tablespoon lime juice
- 1 tablespoon cilantro, chopped

Directions:

1. Heat up a pan with the oil over medium heat, add the onion, chili powder and the rosemary, toss and sauté for 5 minutes.

2. Add the meat, and brown for 5 minutes more.
3. Add the potatoes and the rest of the ingredients except the cilantro, toss gently, bring to a simmer and cook over medium heat for 30 minutes.
4. Divide the mix between plates and serve with the cilantro sprinkled on top.

Nutrition info per serving: 149 calories, 4.2g protein, 18.5g carbohydrates, 7.5g fat, 4.5g fiber, 0mg cholesterol, 90mg sodium, 571mg potassium

Chicken and Greens

Preparation time: 10 minutes

Cooking time: 25 minutes

Servings: 4

Ingredients:

- 2 chicken breasts, skinless, boneless and cubed
- 3 cups mustard greens
- 1 cup canned tomatoes, no-salt-added, chopped
- 1 red onion, chopped
- 2 tablespoons avocado oil
- 1 teaspoon oregano, dried
- 2 garlic cloves, minced
- 1 tablespoon chives, chopped
- 1 tablespoon balsamic vinegar
- A pinch of black pepper

Directions:

1. Heat up a pan with the oil over medium-high heat, add the onion and the garlic and sauté for 5 minutes.
2. Add the meat and brown it for 5 minutes more.

3. Add the greens, tomatoes and the other ingredients, toss, cook for 20 minutes over medium heat, divide between plates and serve.

Nutrition info per serving: 281 calories, 38.2g protein, 7.6g carbohydrates, 10.4g fat, 3g fiber, 111mg cholesterol, 132mg sodium, 639mg potassium

Herbed Chicken Mix

Preparation time: 10 minutes

Cooking time: 50 minutes

Servings: 4

Ingredients:

- 2 pounds chicken thighs, boneless and skinless
- 2 tablespoons olive oil
- 2 red onions, sliced
- A pinch of black pepper
- 1 teaspoon thyme, dried
- 1 teaspoon basil, dried
- 1 cup green apples, cored and roughly cubed
- 2 garlic cloves, minced
- 2 cups low-sodium chicken stock
- 1 tablespoon lemon juice
- 1 cup tomatoes, cubed
- 1 tablespoon cilantro, chopped

Directions:

1. Heat up a pan with the oil over medium-high heat, add the onions and garlic, and sauté for 5 minutes.
2. Add the chicken and brown for another 5 minutes.
3. Add the thyme, basil and the other ingredients, toss gently, introduce in the oven and bake at 390 degrees F for 40 minutes.
4. Divide the chicken and apples mix between plates and serve.

Nutrition info per serving: 557 calories, 67.4g protein, 15.4g carbohydrates, 24.1g fat, 3.2g fiber, 202mg cholesterol, 269mg sodium, 813mg potassium

Cumin Chicken

Preparation time: 10 minutes

Cooking time: 1 hour

Servings: 6

Ingredients:

- 2 pounds chicken thighs, boneless and skinless
- 1 yellow onion, chopped
- 2 tablespoons olive oil
- 3 garlic cloves, minced
- 1 tablespoon coriander seeds, ground
- 1 teaspoon cumin, ground
- 1 cup low-sodium chicken stock
- 4 tablespoons chipotle chili paste
- A pinch of black pepper
- 1 tablespoon coriander, chopped

Directions:

1. Heat up a pan with the oil over medium heat, add the onion and the garlic and sauté for 5 minutes.
2. Add the meat and brown for 5 minutes more.

3. Add the rest of the ingredients, toss, introduce everything in the oven and bake at 390 degrees F for 50 minutes.
4. Divide the whole mix between plates and serve.

Nutrition info per serving: 372 calories, 44.9g protein, 6.4g carbohydrates, 17.6g fat, 0.5g fiber, 138mg cholesterol, 274mg sodium, 407mg potassium

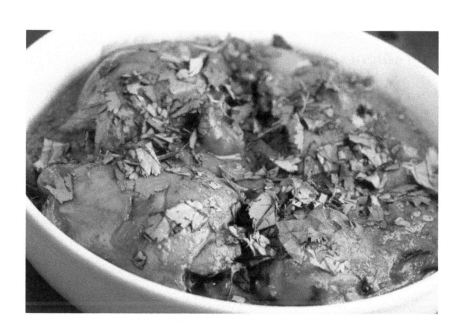

Oregano Turkey and Tomato Mix

Preparation time: 10 minutes

Cooking time: 35 minutes

Servings: 4

Ingredients:

- 1 big turkey breast, boneless, skinless and sliced
- 1 tablespoon chives, chopped
- 1 tablespoon oregano, chopped
- 1 tablespoon basil, chopped
- 1 tablespoon coriander, chopped
- 2 shallots, chopped
- 2 tablespoons olive oil
- 1 cup low-sodium chicken stock
- 1 cup tomatoes, cubed
- Salt and black pepper to the taste

Directions:

1. Heat up a pan with the oil over medium heat, add the shallots and the meat and brown for 5 minutes.

2. Add the chives and the other ingredients, toss, bring to a simmer and cook over medium heat for 30 minutes.
3. Divide the mix between plates and serve.

Nutrition info per serving: 189 calories, 14.5g protein, 11.1g carbohydrates, 10.2g fat, 1.5g fiber, 55mg cholesterol, 1237mg sodium, 497mg potassium

Ginger Chicken

Preparation time: 10 minutes

Cooking time: 35 minutes

Servings: 4

Ingredients:

- 1 pound chicken breast, skinless, boneless and cubed
- 1 tablespoon ginger, grated
- 1 tablespoon olive oil
- 2 shallots, chopped
- 1 tablespoon balsamic vinegar
- A pinch of black pepper
- ¾ cup low-sodium chicken stock
- 1 tablespoon basil, chopped

Directions:

1. Heat up a pan with the oil over medium heat, add the shallots and the ginger, stir and sauté for 5 minutes.
2. Add the rest of the ingredients except the chicken, toss, bring to a simmer and cook for 5 minutes more.

3. Add the chicken, toss, simmer the whole mix for 25 minutes, divide between plates and serve.

Nutrition info per serving: 169 calories, 24.5g protein, 1.9g carbohydrates, 6.4g fat, 0.2g fiber, 73mg cholesterol, 84mg sodium, 459mg potassium

Chicken and Green Onions

Preparation time: 10 minutes

Cooking time: 35 minutes

Servings: 4

Ingredients:

- 2 pounds chicken breast, skinless, boneless and halved
- 2 cups corn
- 2 tablespoons avocado oil
- A pinch of black pepper
- 1 teaspoon smoked paprika
- 1 bunch green onions, chopped
- 1 cup low-sodium chicken stock

Directions:

1. Heat up a pan with the oil over medium-high heat, add the green onions, stir and sauté them for 5 minutes.
2. Add the chicken and brown it for 5 minutes more.

3. Add the corn and the other ingredients, toss, introduce the pan in the oven and cook at 390 degrees F for 25 minutes.
4. Divide the mix between plates and serve.

Nutrition info per serving: 338 calories, 51.1g protein, 15.5g carbohydrates, 7.5g fat, 2.7g fiber, 145mg cholesterol, 162mg sodium, 1092mg potassium

Parsley Turkey and Quinoa

Preparation time: 10 minutes

Cooking time: 40 minutes

Servings: 4

Ingredients:

- 1 pound turkey breast, skinless, boneless and cubed
- 1 tablespoon olive oil
- 1 cup quinoa
- 2 cups low-sodium chicken stock
- 1 tablespoon lime juice
- 1 tablespoon parsley, chopped
- A pinch of black pepper
- 1 tablespoon red curry paste

Directions:

1. Heat up a pan with the oil over medium-high heat, add the meat and brown it for 5 minutes.

2. Add the quinoa and the rest of the ingredients, toss, bring to a simmer and cook over medium heat for 35 minutes.
3. Divide everything between plates and serve.

Nutrition info per serving: 322 calories, 25.9g protein, 32.9g carbohydrates, 9.1g fat, 3.6g fiber, 49mg cholesterol, 1416mg sodium, 587mg potassium

Turkey and Parsnips

Preparation time: 10 minutes

Cooking time: 40 minutes

Servings: 4

Ingredients:

- 1 pound turkey breast, skinless, boneless and cubed
- 2 parsnips, peeled and cubed
- 2 teaspoons cumin, ground
- 1 tablespoon parsley, chopped
- 2 tablespoons avocado oil
- 2 shallots, chopped
- 1 cup low-sodium chicken stock
- 4 garlic cloves, minced
- A pinch of black pepper

Directions:

1. Heat up a pan with the oil over medium heat, add the shallots and the garlic and sauté for 5 minutes.
2. Add the turkey, toss and cook for 5 minutes more.

3. Add the parsnips and the other ingredients, toss, simmer over medium heat for 30 minutes more, divide between plates and serve.

Nutrition info per serving: 166 calories, 20.6g protein, 13.5g carbohydrates, 3.1g fat, 2.7g fiber, 49mg cholesterol, 1192mg sodium, 542mg potassium

Turkey and Chickpeas

Preparation time: 10 minutes

Cooking time: 40 minutes

Servings: 4

Ingredients:

- 1 cup canned chickpeas, no-salt-added, drained
- 1 cup low-sodium chicken stock
- 1 pound turkey breast, skinless, boneless and cubed
- A pinch of black pepper
- 1 teaspoon oregano, dried
- 1 teaspoon nutmeg, ground
- 2 tablespoons olive oil
- 1 yellow onion, chopped
- 1 green bell pepper, chopped
- 1 cup cilantro, chopped

Directions:

1. Heat up a pan with the oil over medium heat, add the onion, bell pepper and the meat and cook for 10 minutes stirring often.

2. Add the rest of the ingredients, toss, bring to a simmer and cook over medium heat for 30 minutes.
3. Divide the mix between plates and serve.

Nutrition info per serving: 387 calories, 30g protein, 40.6g carbohydrates, 12.3g fat, 10.6g fiber, 49mg cholesterol, 1201mg sodium, 905mg potassium

Turkey and Lentils

Preparation time: 10 minutes

Cooking time: 40 minutes

Servings: 4

Ingredients:

- 2 pounds turkey breast, skinless, boneless and cubed
- 1 cup canned lentils, no-salt-added, drained and rinsed
- 1 tablespoon green curry paste
- 1 teaspoon garam masala
- 2 tablespoons olive oil
- 1 yellow onion, chopped
- 1 garlic clove, minced
- A pinch of black pepper
- 1 tablespoon cilantro, chopped

Directions:

1. Heat up a pan with the oil over medium heat, add the onion, garlic and the meat and brown for 5 minutes stirring often.
2. Add the lentils and the other ingredients, bring to a simmer and cook over medium heat for 35 minutes.
3. Divide the mix between plates and serve.

Nutrition info per serving: 224 calories, 19.8g protein, 16.9g carbohydrates, 8.9g fat, 5g fiber, 38mg cholesterol, 941mg sodium, 491mg potassium

Turkey and Olives

Preparation time: 10 minutes

Cooking time: 35 minutes

Servings: 4

Ingredients:

- 1 cup black beans, no-salt-added and drained
- 1 cup green olives, pitted and halved
- 1 pound turkey breast, skinless, boneless and sliced
- 1 tablespoon cilantro, chopped
- 1 cup tomato sauce, no-salt-added
- 1 tablespoon olive oil

Directions:

1. Grease a baking dish with the oil, arrange the turkey slices inside, add the other ingredients as well, introduce in the oven and bake at 380 degrees F for 35 minutes.
2. Divide between plates and serve.

Nutrition info per serving: 291 calories, 25.6g protein, 24g carbohydrates, 10.1g fat, 6.8g fiber, 49mg cholesterol, 1405mg sodium, 546mg potassium

Rosemary Chicken and Quinoa

Preparation time: 10 minutes

Cooking time: 35 minutes

Servings: 8

Ingredients:

- 1 tablespoon olive oil
- 2 pounds chicken breasts, skinless, boneless and halved
- 1 teaspoon rosemary, ground
- A pinch of salt and black pepper
- 2 shallots, chopped
- 3 tablespoons low-sodium tomato sauce
- 2 cups quinoa, already cooked

Directions:

1. Heat up a pan with the oil over medium-high heat, add the meat and shallots and brown for 2 minutes on each side.

2. Add the rosemary and the other ingredients, toss, introduce in the oven and cook at 370 degrees F for 30 minutes.
3. Divide the mix between plates and serve.

Nutrition info per serving: 39 calories, 39g protein, 28.1g carbohydrates, 12.8g fat, 3.1g fiber, 101mg cholesterol, 130mg sodium, 544mg potassium

Garlic Chicken Wings

Preparation time: 10 minutes

Cooking time: 20 minutes

Servings: 4

Ingredients:

- 2 pounds chicken wings

- 2 teaspoons allspice, ground

- 2 tablespoons avocado oil

- 5 garlic cloves, minced

- Black pepper to the taste

- 2 tablespoons chives, chopped

Directions:

1. In a bowl, combine the chicken wings with the allspice and the other ingredients and toss well.
2. Arrange the chicken wings in a roasting pan and bake at 400 degrees F for 20 minutes.
3. Divide the chicken wings between plates and serve.

Nutrition info per serving: 449 calories, 66.1g protein, 2.4g carbohydrates, 17.8g fat, 0.6g fiber, 202mg cholesterol, 197mg sodium, 603mg potassium

Parsley Chicken and Peas

Preparation time: 10 minutes

Cooking time: 30 minutes

Servings: 4

Ingredients:

- 2 pounds chicken breasts, skinless, boneless and cubed
- 2 cups snow peas
- 2 tablespoons olive oil
- 1 red onion, chopped
- 1 cup canned tomato sauce, no-salt-added
- 2 tablespoons parsley, chopped
- A pinch of black pepper

Directions:

1. Heat up a pan with the oil over medium heat, add the onion and the meat and brown for 5 minutes.

2. Add the peas and the rest of the ingredients, bring to a simmer and cook over medium heat for 25 minutes.
3. Divide the mix between plates and serve.

Nutrition info per serving: 551 calories, 69.4g protein, 2.4g carbohydrates, 11.6g fat, 24.2g fiber, 202mg cholesterol, 521mg sodium, 997mg potassium

Turkey and Broccoli

Preparation time: 10 minutes

Cooking time: 30 minutes

Servings: 4

Ingredients:

- 1 red onion, chopped

- 1 pound turkey breast, skinless, boneless and cubed

- 2 cups broccoli florets

- 1 teaspoon cumin, ground

- 3 garlic cloves, minced

- 2 tablespoons olive oil

- 14 ounces coconut milk

- A pinch of black pepper

- ¼ cup cilantro, chopped

Directions:

1. Heat up a pot with the oil over medium heat, add the onion and the garlic, stir and sauté for 5 minutes.
2. Add the turkey, toss and brown for 5 minutes.
3. Add the broccoli and the rest of the ingredients, bring to a simmer over medium heat and cook for 20 minutes.
4. Divide the mix between plates and serve.

Nutrition info per serving: 438 calories, 23.5g protein, 16.9g carbohydrates, 32.9g fat, 4.7g fiber, 49mg cholesterol, 1184mg sodium, 811mg potassium

Paprika Chicken

Preparation time: 10 minutes

Cooking time: 30 minutes

Servings: 4

Ingredients:

- 1 pound chicken breast, skinless, boneless and cubed
- 1 cup low-sodium chicken stock
- 1 tablespoon avocado oil
- 2 teaspoons cloves, ground
- 1 yellow onion, chopped
- 2 teaspoons sweet paprika
- 3 tomatoes, cubed
- A pinch of salt and black pepper
- ½ cup parsley, chopped

Directions:

1. Heat up a pan with the oil over medium heat, add the onion and sauté for 5 minutes.
2. Add the chicken and brown for 5 minutes more.

3. Add the stock and the rest of the ingredients, bring to a simmer and cook over medium heat for 20 minutes more.
4. Divide the mix between plates and serve.

Nutrition info per serving: 172 calories, 25.9g protein, 8.1g carbohydrates, 3.9g fat, 2.9g fiber, 73mg cholesterol, 104mg sodium, 767mg potassium

Chicken and Artichokes

Preparation time: 10 minutes

Cooking time: 30 minutes

Servings: 4

Ingredients:

- 2 chicken breasts, skinless, boneless and halved
- 1 tablespoon ginger, grated
- 1 cup canned tomatoes, no-salt-added, chopped
- 10 ounces canned artichokes, no-salt-added, drained and quartered
- 2 tablespoons lemon juice
- 2 tablespoons olive oil
- A pinch of black pepper

Directions:

1. Heat up a pan with the oil over medium heat, add the ginger and the artichokes, toss and cook for 5 minutes.
2. Add the chicken and cook for 5 minutes more.

3. Add the rest of the ingredients, bring to a simmer and cook for 20 minutes more.
4. Divide everything between plates and serve.

Nutrition info per serving: 247 calories, 24g protein, 10.3g carbohydrates, 12.8g fat, 4.6g fiber, 65mg cholesterol, 134mg sodium, 574mg potassium

Peppercorn Turkey

Preparation time: 10 minutes

Cooking time: 30 minutes

Servings: 4

Ingredients:

- ½ tablespoon black peppercorns
- 1 tablespoon olive oil
- 1 pound turkey breast, skinless, boneless and cubed
- 1 cup low-sodium chicken stock
- 3 garlic cloves, minced
- 2 tomatoes, cubed
- A pinch of black pepper
- 2 tablespoons spring onions, chopped

Directions:

1. Heat up a pan with the oil over medium heat, add the garlic and the turkey and brown for 5 minutes.
2. Add the peppercorns and the rest of the ingredients, bring to a simmer and cook over medium heat for 25 minutes.
3. Divide the mix between plates and serve.

Nutrition info per serving: 167 calories, 20.4g protein, 8.6g carbohydrates, 5.6g fat, 1.7g fiber, 49mg cholesterol, 1189mg sodium, 516mg potassium

Chicken and Veggies

Preparation time: 10 minutes

Cooking time: 40 minutes

Servings: 4

Ingredients:

- 2 pounds chicken breasts, skinless, boneless and cubed
- 1 carrot, cubed
- 1 celery stalk, chopped
- 1 tomato, cubed
- 2 small red onions, sliced
- 1 zucchini, cubed
- 2 garlic cloves, minced
- 1 tablespoon rosemary, chopped
- 2 tablespoons olive oil
- Black pepper to the taste
- ½ cup low-sodium vegetable stock

Directions:

1. Heat up a pan with the oil over medium heat, add the onions and the garlic, stir and sauté for 5 minutes.

2. Add the chicken, toss and brown it for 5 minutes more.
3. Add the carrot and the other ingredients, toss, bring to a simmer and cook over medium heat for 30 minutes.
4. Divide the mix between plates and serve.

Nutrition info per serving: 530 calories, 67.2g protein, 8.7g carbohydrates, 24.1g fat, 2.4g fiber, 202mg cholesterol, 234mg sodium, 857mg potassium

Chicken and Cabbage

Preparation time: 10 minutes

Cooking time: 25 minutes

Servings: 4

Ingredients:

- 1 pound chicken breast, skinless, boneless and cubed
- 2 tablespoons olive oil
- 2 carrots, peeled and grated
- 1 teaspoon sweet paprika
- ½ cup low-sodium vegetable stock
- 1 red cabbage head, shredded
- 1 yellow onion, chopped
- Black pepper to the taste

Directions:

1. Heat up a pan with the oil over medium heat, add the onion, stir and sauté for 5 minutes.

2. Add the meat, and brown it for 5 minutes more.

3. Add the carrots and the other ingredients, toss, bring to a simmer and cook over medium heat for 15 minutes.

4. Divide everything between plates and serve.

Nutrition info per serving: 261 calories, 27.1g protein, 16.7g carbohydrates, 10.1g fat, 6.1g fiber, 73mg cholesterol, 130mg sodium, 889mg potassium

Pumpkin Seeds Bowls

Preparation time: 10 minutes

Cooking time: 2 hours

Servings: 4

Ingredients:

- Cooking spray
- 2 teaspoons nutmeg, ground
- 1 cup pumpkin seeds
- 2 apples, cored and thinly sliced

Directions:

1. Arrange the pumpkin seeds and the apple chips on a lined baking sheet, sprinkle the nutmeg all over, grease them with the spray, introduce in the oven and bake at 300 degrees F for 2 hours.
2. Divide into bowls and serve as a snack.

Nutrition info per serving: 250 calories, 8.8g protein, 22.1g carbohydrates, 16.4g fat, 4.3g fiber, 0mg cholesterol, 7mg sodium, 402mg potassium

Yogurt Dip

Preparation time: 5 minutes

Cooking time: 0 minutes

Servings: 4

Ingredients:

- 2 cups fat-free Greek yogurt

- 1 tablespoon parsley, chopped

- ¼ cup canned tomatoes, no-salt-added, chopped

- 2 tablespoons chives, chopped

- Black pepper to the taste

Directions:

1. In a bowl, mix the yogurt with the parsley and the other ingredients, whisk well, divide into small bowls and serve as a party dip.

Nutrition info per serving: 53 calories, 5.2g protein, 7.6g carbohydrates, 0g fat, 0.2g fiber, 3mg cholesterol, 41mg sodium, 36mg potassium

Rosemary Beet Bites

Preparation time: 10 minutes

Cooking time: 35 minutes

Servings: 2

Ingredients:

- 1 teaspoon cayenne pepper
- 2 beets, peeled and cubed
- 1 teaspoon rosemary, dried
- 1 tablespoon olive oil
- 2 teaspoons lime juice

Directions:

1. In a roasting pan, combine the beet bites with the cayenne and the other ingredients, toss, introduce in the oven, roast at 355 degrees F for 35 minutes, divide into small bowls and serve as a snack.

Nutrition info per serving: 109 calories, 1.8g protein, 10.9g carbohydrates, 7.4g fat, 2.5g fiber, 0mg cholesterol, 78mg sodium, 329mg potassium

Pecans Bowls

Preparation time: 10 minutes

Cooking time: 10 minutes

Servings: 4

Ingredients:

- 2 cup walnuts
- 1 cup pecans, chopped
- 1 teaspoon avocado oil
- ½ teaspoon sweet paprika

Directions:

1. Spread the grapes and pecans on a lined baking sheet, add the oil and the paprika, toss, and bake at 400 degrees F for 10 minutes.
2. Divide into bowls and serve as a snack.

Nutrition info per serving: 584 calories, 18.1g protein, 10.4g carbohydrates, 57.1g fat, 7.4g fiber, 0mg cholesterol, 1mg sodium, 453mg potassium

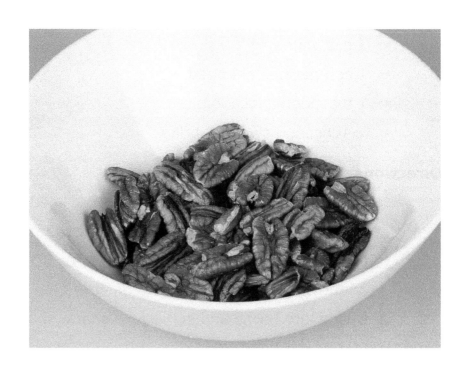

Salmon Muffins

Preparation time: 10 minutes

Cooking time: 25 minutes

Servings: 4

Ingredients:

- 1 cup low-fat mozzarella cheese, shredded
- 8 ounces smoked salmon, skinless, boneless, and chopped
- 1 cup almond flour
- 1 egg, whisked
- 1 teaspoon parsley, dried
- 1 garlic clove, minced
- Black pepper to the taste
- Cooking spray

Directions:

1. In a bowl, combine the salmon with the mozzarella and the other ingredients except the cooking spray and stir well.

2. Divide this mix into a muffin tray greased with the cooking spray, bake in the oven at 375 degrees F for 25 minutes and serve as a snack.

Nutrition info per serving: 163 calories, 21.3g protein, 2.9g carbohydrates, 7g fat, 1.8g fiber, 59mg cholesterol, 1392mg sodium, 119mg potassium

Squash Bites

Preparation time: 10 minutes

Cooking time: 20 minutes

Servings: 8

Ingredients:

- A drizzle of olive oil

- 1 big butternut squash, peeled and minced

- 2 tablespoons cilantro, chopped

- 2 eggs, whisked

- ½ cup whole wheat flour

- Black pepper to the taste

- 2 shallots, chopped

- 2 garlic cloves, minced

Directions:

1. In a bowl, mix the squash with the cilantro and the other ingredients except the oil, stir well and shape medium balls out of this mix.

2. Arrange them on a lined baking sheet, grease them with the oil, bake at 400 degrees F for 10 minutes on each side, divide into bowls and serve.

Nutrition info per serving: 79 calories, 3g protein, 14.9g carbohydrates, 1.2g fat, 1.6g fiber, 41mg cholesterol, 19mg sodium, 282mg potassium

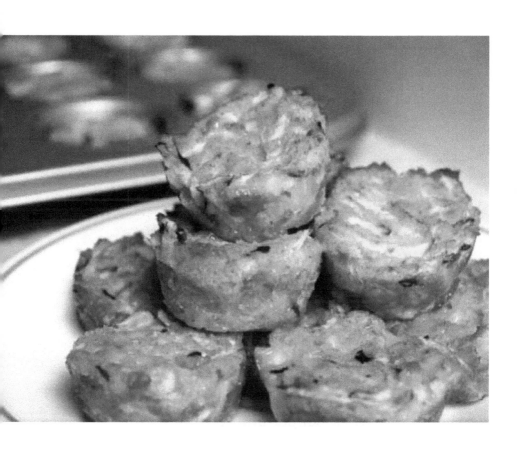

Pearl Onions Snack

Preparation time: 10 minutes

Cooking time: 30 minutes

Servings: 8

Ingredients:

- 20 white pearl onions, peeled

- 3 tablespoons parsley, chopped

- 1 tablespoon chives, chopped

- Black pepper to the taste

- 1 cup low-fat mozzarella, grated

- 1 tablespoon olive oil

Directions:

1. Spread the pearl onions on a lined baking sheet, add the oil, parsley, chives and the black pepper and toss.
2. Sprinkle the mozzarella on top, bake at 390 degrees F for 30 minutes, divide into bowls and serve cold as a snack.

Nutrition info per serving: 171 calories, 6.1g protein, 26.2g carbohydrates, 5.5g fat, 6g fiber, 13mg cholesterol, 71mg sodium, 421mg potassium

Oregano Broccoli Bars

Preparation time: 10 minutes

Cooking time: 25 minutes

Servings: 8

Ingredients:

- 1 pound broccoli florets, chopped
- ½ cup low-fat mozzarella cheese, shredded
- 2 eggs, whisked
- 1 teaspoon oregano, dried
- 1 teaspoon basil, dried
- Black pepper to the taste

Directions:

1. In a bowl, mix the broccoli with the cheese and the other ingredients, stir well, spread into a rectangle pan and press well on the bottom.
2. Introduce in the oven at 380 degrees F, bake for 25 minutes, cut into bars and serve cold.

Nutrition info per serving: 56 calories, 7g protein, 4.5g carbohydrates, 1.3g fat, 2.1g fiber, 43mg cholesterol, 154mg sodium, 198mg potassium

Pineapple Salsa

Preparation time: 10 minutes

Cooking time: 40 minutes

Servings: 4

Ingredients:

- 20 ounces canned pineapple, drained and cubed
- 1 cup sun-dried tomatoes, cubed
- 1 tablespoon basil, chopped
- 1 tablespoon avocado oil
- 1 teaspoon lime juice
- 1 cup black olives, pitted and sliced
- Black pepper to the taste

Directions:

1. In a bowl, combine the pineapple cubes with the tomatoes and the other ingredients, toss, divide into smaller cups and serve as a snack.

Nutrition info per serving: 122 calories, 1.5g protein, 22.7g carbohydrates, 4.3g fat, 3.8g fiber, 0mg cholesterol, 297mg sodium, 277mg potassium

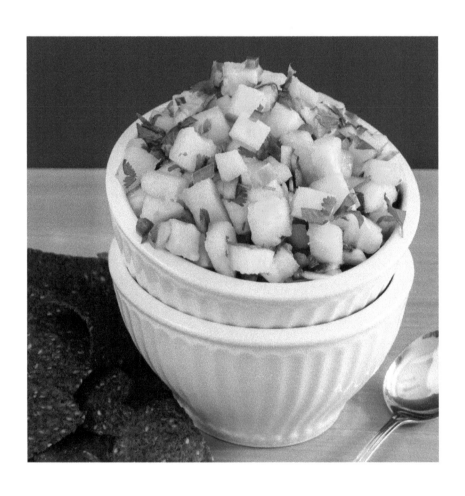

Creamy Turkey Mix

Preparation time: 5 minutes

Cooking time: 25 minutes

Servings: 4

Ingredients:

- 2 tablespoons olive oil

- 1 turkey breast, skinless, boneless and sliced

- A pinch of black pepper

- 1 tablespoon basil, chopped

- 3 garlic cloves, minced

- 14 ounces canned artichokes, no-salt-added, chopped

- 1 cup coconut cream

- ¾ cup low-fat mozzarella, shredded

Directions:

1. Heat up a pan with the oil over medium-high heat, add the meat, garlic and the black pepper, toss and cook for 5 minutes.

2. Add the rest of the ingredients except the cheese, toss and cook over medium heat for 15 minutes.
3. Sprinkle the cheese, cook everything for 5 minutes more, divide between plates and serve.

Nutrition info per serving: 268 calories, 8.8g protein, 15g carbohydrates, 21.5g fat, 7.3g fiber, 3mg cholesterol, 225mg sodium, 537mg potassium

Turkey and Onion Mix

Preparation time: 10 minutes

Cooking time: 30 minutes

Servings: 4

Ingredients:

- 2 tablespoons avocado oil

- 1 red onion, chopped

- 2 garlic cloves, minced

- A pinch of black pepper

- 1 tablespoon oregano, chopped

- 1 big turkey breast, skinless, boneless and cubed

- 1 and ½ cups low-sodium beef stock

- 1 tablespoon chives, chopped

Directions:

1. Heat up a pan with the oil over medium heat, add the onion, stir and sauté for 3 minutes.

2. Add the garlic and the meat, toss and cook for 3 minutes more.
3. Add the rest of the ingredients, toss, simmer everything over medium heat for 25 minutes, divide between plates and serve.

Nutrition info per serving: 32 calories, 1.4g protein, 4.6g carbohydrates, 1.1g fat, 1.4g fiber, 0mg cholesterol, 154mg sodium, 90mg potassium

Balsamic Chicken

Preparation time: 10 minutes

Cooking time: 35 minutes

Servings: 4

Ingredients:

- 1 tablespoon avocado oil

- 1 pound chicken breast, skinless, boneless and halved

- 2 garlic cloves, minced

- 2 shallots, chopped

- ½ cup orange juice

- 1 tablespoon orange zest, grated

- 3 tablespoons balsamic vinegar

- 1 teaspoon rosemary, chopped

Directions:

1. Heat up a pan with the oil over medium-high heat, add the shallots and the garlic, toss and sauté for 2 minutes.

2. Add the meat, toss gently and cook for 3 minutes more.
3. Add the rest of the ingredients, toss, introduce the pan in the oven and bake at 340 degrees F for 30 minutes.
4. Divide between plates and serve.

Nutrition info per serving: 159 calories, 24.6g protein, 5.4g carbohydrates, 3.4g fat, 0.5g fiber, 73mg cholesterol, 60mg sodium, 530mg potassium

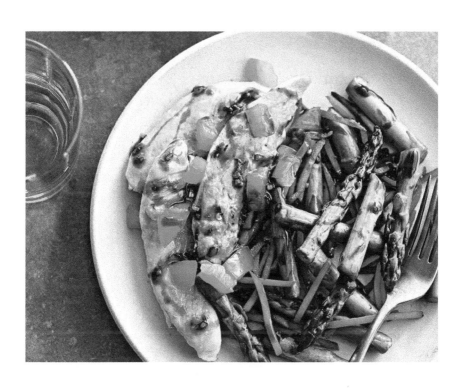

Turkey and Garlic Sauce

Preparation time: 10 minutes

Cooking time: 40 minutes

Servings: 4

Ingredients:

- 1 turkey breast, boneless, skinless and cubed
- ½ pound white mushrooms, halved
- 1/3 cup coconut aminos
- 2 garlic cloves, minced
- 2 tablespoons olive oil
- A pinch of black pepper
- 2 green onion, chopped
- 3 tablespoons garlic sauce
- 1 tablespoon rosemary, chopped

Directions:

1. Heat up a pan with the oil over medium heat, add the green onions, garlic sauce and the garlic and sauté for 5 minutes.
2. Add the meat and brown it for 5 minutes more.
3. Add the rest of the ingredients, introduce in the oven and bake at 390 degrees F for 30 minutes.
4. Divide the mix between plates and serve.

Nutrition info per serving: 100 calories, 2.1g protein, 7.5g carbohydrates, 7.3g fat, 1.2g fiber, 0mg cholesterol, 30mg sodium, 216mg potassium

Coconut Chicken and Olives

Preparation time: 10 minutes

Cooking time: 25 minutes

Servings: 4

Ingredients:

- 1 pound chicken breasts, skinless, boneless and roughly cubed
- A pinch of black pepper
- 1 tablespoon avocado oil
- 1 red onion, chopped
- 1 cup coconut milk
- 1 tablespoon lemon juice
- 1 cup kalamata olives, pitted and sliced
- ¼ cup cilantro, chopped

Directions:

1. Heat up a pan with the oil over medium-high heat, add the onion and the meat and brown for 5 minutes.
2. Add the rest of the ingredients, toss, bring to a simmer and cook over medium heat for 20 minutes more.
3. Divide between plates and serve.

Nutrition info per serving: 409 calories, 34.9g protein, 8.3g carbohydrates, 26.8g fat, 3.2g fiber, 101mg cholesterol, 402mg sodium, 497mg potassium

Turkey and Peach

Preparation time: 10 minutes

Cooking time: 25 minutes

Servings: 4

Ingredients:

- 1 tablespoon avocado oil

- 1 turkey breast, skinless, boneless and sliced

- A pinch of black pepper

- 1 yellow onion, chopped

- 4 peaches, stones removed and cut into wedges

- ¼ cup balsamic vinegar

- 2 tablespoons chives, chopped

Directions:

1. Heat up a pan with the oil over medium-high heat, add the meat and the onion, toss and brown for 5 minutes.

2. Add the rest of the ingredients except the chives, toss gently and bake at 390 degrees F for 20 minutes.
3. Divide everything between plates and serve with the chives sprinkled on top.

Nutrition info per serving: 79 calories, 1.8g protein, 17g carbohydrates, 0.9g fat, 3.1g fiber, 0mg cholesterol, 5mg sodium, 352mg potassium

Paprika Chicken and Spinach

Preparation time: 10 minutes

Cooking time: 25 minutes

Servings: 4

Ingredients:

- 1 tablespoon avocado oil

- 1 pound chicken breast, skinless, boneless and cubed

- ½ teaspoon basil, dried

- A pinch of black pepper

- ¼ cup low-sodium vegetable stock

- 2 cups baby spinach

- 2 shallots, chopped

- 2 garlic cloves, minced

- ½ teaspoon sweet paprika

- 2/3 cup coconut cream

- 2 tablespoons cilantro, chopped

Directions:

1. Heat up a pan with the oil over medium-high heat, add the meat, basil, black pepper and brown for 5 minutes.
2. Add the shallots and the garlic and cook for another 5 minutes.
3. Add the rest of the ingredients, toss, bring to a simmer and cook over medium heat fro 15 minutes more.
4. Divide between plates and serve hot.

Nutrition info per serving: 237 calories, 25.8g protein, 4.5g carbohydrates, 12.9g fat, 1.5g fiber, 73mg cholesterol, 81mg sodium, 652mg potassium

Chicken and Tomatoes Mix

Preparation time: 10 minutes

Cooking time: 25 minutes

Servings: 4

Ingredients:

- 2 chicken breasts, skinless, boneless and cubed

- 2 tablespoons avocado oil

- 2 spring onions, chopped

- 1 bunch asparagus, trimmed and halved

- ½ teaspoon sweet paprika

- A pinch of black pepper

- 14 ounces canned tomatoes, no-salt-added, drained and chopped

Directions:

1. Heat up a pan with the oil over medium-high heat, add the meat and the spring onions, stir and cook for 5 minutes.
2. Add the asparagus and the other ingredients, toss, cover the pan and cook over medium heat for 20 minutes.
3. Divide everything between plates and serve.

Nutrition info per serving: 38 calories, 2g protein, 6.2g carbohydrates, 1.2g fat, 2.5g fiber, 0mg cholesterol, 8mg sodium, 353mg potassium

Basil Turkey and Broccoli

Preparation time: 10 minutes

Cooking time: 25 minutes

Servings: 4

Ingredients:

- 1 tablespoon olive oil

- 1 big turkey breast, skinless, boneless and cubed

- 2 cups broccoli florets

- 2 shallots, chopped

- 2 garlic cloves, minced

- 1 tablespoon basil, chopped

- 1 tablespoon cilantro, chopped

- ½ cup coconut cream

Directions:

1. Heat up a pan with the oil over medium-high heat, add the meat, shallots and the garlic, toss and brown for 5 minutes.
2. Add the broccoli and the other ingredients, toss everything, cook for 20 minutes over medium heat, divide between plates and serve.

Nutrition info per serving: 121 calories, 2.3g protein, 6.1g carbohydrates, 10.8g fat, 1.9g fiber, 0mg cholesterol, 23mg sodium, 250mg potassium

Chicken with Green Beans and Sauce

Preparation time: 10 minutes

Cooking time: 25 minutes

Servings: 4

Ingredients:

- 2 tablespoons olive oil

- 10 ounces green beans, trimmed and halved

- 1 yellow onion, chopped

- 1 tablespoon dill, chopped

- 2 chicken breasts, skinless, boneless and halved

- 2 cups tomato sauce, no-salt-added

- ½ teaspoon red pepper flakes, crushed

Directions:

1. Heat up a pan with the oil over medium-high heat, add the onion and the meat and brown it for 2 minutes on each side.
2. Add the green beans and the other ingredients, toss, introduce in the oven and bake at 380 degrees F for 20 minutes.
3. Divide between plates and serve right away.

Nutrition info per serving: 126 calories, 3.5g protein, 14.8g carbohydrates, 7.5g fat, 5g fiber, 0mg cholesterol, 649mg sodium, 625mg potassium

Chicken with Zucchini

Preparation time: 5 minutes

Cooking time: 25 minutes

Servings: 4

Ingredients:

- 1 pound chicken breasts, skinless, boneless and cubed
- 1 cup low-sodium chicken stock
- 2 zucchinis, roughly cubed
- 1 tablespoon olive oil
- 1 cup canned tomatoes, no-salt-added, chopped
- 1 yellow onion, chopped
- 1 teaspoon chili powder
- 1 tablespoon cilantro, chopped

Directions:

1. Heat up a pan with the oil over medium-high heat, add the meat and the onion, toss and brown for 5 minutes.

2. Add the zucchinis and the rest of the ingredients, toss gently, reduce the heat to medium and cook for 20 minutes.
3. Divide everything between plates and serve.

Nutrition info per serving: 284 calories, 35g protein, 14.8g carbohydrates, 8g fat, 12.3g fiber, 2.4mg cholesterol, 151mg sodium, 693mg potassium

Lemon Chicken Mix

Preparation time: 10 minutes

Cooking time: 20 minutes

Servings: 4

Ingredients:

- 2 chicken breasts, skinless, boneless and halved
- Juice of ½ lemon
- 2 tablespoons olive oil
- 2 garlic cloves, minced
- ½ cup low-sodium vegetable stock
- 1 avocado, peeled, pitted and cut into wedges
- A pinch of black pepper

Directions:

1. Heat up a pan with the oil over medium heat, add the garlic and the meat and brown for 2 minutes on each side.

2. Add the lemon juice and the other ingredients, bring to a simmer and cook over medium heat for 15 minutes.
3. Divide the whole mix between plates and serve.

Nutrition info per serving: 170 calories, 1.4g protein, 6g carbohydrates, 16.9g fat, 3.7g fiber, 0mg cholesterol, 21mg sodium, 277mg potassium

Ginger Turkey Mix

Preparation time: 10 minutes

Cooking time: 20 minutes

Servings: 4

Ingredients:

- 1 turkey breast, boneless, skinless and roughly cubed
- 2 scallions, chopped
- 1 pound bok choy, torn
- 2 tablespoons olive oil
- ½ teaspoon ginger, grated
- A pinch of black pepper
- ½ cup low-sodium vegetable stock

Directions:

1. Heat up a pot with the oil over medium-high heat, add the scallions and the ginger and sauté for 2 minutes.
2. Add the meat and brown for 5 minutes more.

3. Add the rest of the ingredients, toss, simmer for 13 minutes more, divide between plates and serve.

Nutrition info per serving: 81 calories, 2g protein, 3.7g carbohydrates, 7.3g fat, 1.5g fiber, 0mg cholesterol, 95mg sodium, 327mg potassium

Chives Chicken

Preparation time: 10 minutes

Cooking time: 25 minutes

Servings: 4

Ingredients:

- 2 chicken breasts, skinless, boneless and roughly cubed

- 3 red onions, sliced

- 2 tablespoons olive oil

- 1 cup low-sodium vegetable stock

- A pinch of black pepper

- 1 tablespoon cilantro, chopped

- 1 tablespoon chives, chopped

Directions:

1. Heat up a pan with the oil over medium heat, add the onions and a pinch of black pepper, and sauté for 10 minutes stirring often.

2. Add the chicken and cook for 3 minutes more.
3. Add the rest of the ingredients, bring to a simmer and cook over medium heat for 12 minutes more.
4. Divide the chicken and onions mix between plates and serve.

Nutrition info per serving: 99 calories, 1.3g protein, 8.8g carbohydrates, 7.1g fat, 2.1g fiber, 0mg cholesterol, 39mg sodium, 158mg potassium

Turkey with Pepper and Rice

Preparation time: 10 minutes

Cooking time: 42 minutes

Servings: 4

Ingredients:

- 1 turkey breast, skinless, boneless and cubed

- 1 cup brown rice

- 2 cups low-sodium vegetable stock

- 1 teaspoon hot paprika

- 2 small Serrano peppers, chopped

- 2 garlic cloves, minced

- 2 tablespoons olive oil

- ½ red bell pepper chopped

- A pinch of black pepper

Directions:

1. Heat up a pan with the oil over medium heat, add the Serrano peppers and garlic and sauté for 2 minutes.
2. Add the meat and brown it for 5 minutes.
3. Add the rice and the other ingredients, bring to a simmer and cook over medium heat for 35 minutes.
4. Stir, divide between plates and serve.

Nutrition info per serving: 245 calories, 4g protein, 40.2g carbohydrates, 7.3g fat, 1.3g fiber, 0mg cholesterol, 76mg sodium, 134mg potassium

Chicken and Leeks

Preparation time: 10 minutes

Cooking time: 40 minutes

Servings: 4

Ingredients:

- 1 pound chicken breast, skinless, boneless and cubed
- A pinch of black pepper
- 2 tablespoons avocado oil
- 1 tablespoon tomato sauce, no-salt-added
- 1 cup low-sodium vegetable stock
- 4 leek, roughly chopped
- ½ cup lemon juice

Directions:

1. Heat up a pan with the oil over medium heat, add the leeks, toss and sauté for 10 minutes.
2. Add the chicken and the other ingredients, toss, cook over medium heat for 20 minutes more, divide between plates and serve.

Nutrition info per serving: 214 calories, 25.9g protein, 14.7g carbohydrates, 5.1g fat, 2.1g fiber, 73mg cholesterol, 172mg sodium, 652mg potassium

Turkey and Cabbage Mix

Preparation time: 10 minutes

Cooking time: 35 minutes

Servings: 4

Ingredients:

- 1 big turkey breast, skinless, boneless and cubed
- 1 cup low-sodium chicken stock
- 1 tablespoon coconut oil, melted
- 1 Savoy cabbage, shredded
- 1 teaspoon chili powder
- 1 teaspoon sweet paprika
- 1 garlic clove, minced
- 1 yellow onion, chopped

Directions:

1. Heat up a pan with the oil over medium heat, add the meat and brown for 5 minutes.
2. Add the garlic and the onion, toss and sauté for 5 minutes more.

3. Add the cabbage and the other ingredients, toss, bring to a simmer and cook over medium heat for 25 minutes.
4. Divide everything between plates and serve.

Nutrition info per serving: 91 calories, 3.1g protein, 13.8g carbohydrates, 3.8g fat, 5.5g fiber, 0mg cholesterol, 76mg sodium, 372mg potassium

Lightning Source UK Ltd.
Milton Keynes UK
UKHW020856160621
385598UK00001B/62